T0018250

THINGS TO DO

WHEN YOU'RE

Feeling Blue

An Hachette UK Company
www.hachette.co.uk

Vie Books, an imprint of Summersdale Publishers Ltd
Part of Octopus Publishing Group Limited
Carmelite House
50 Victoria Embankment
LONDON
EC4Y 0DZ
UK

www.summersdale.com

Printed and bound in China

ISBN: 978-1-80007-158-2

Substantial discounts on bulk quantities of Summersdale books are available to corporations, professional associations and other organizations. For details contact general enquiries: telephone: +44 (0) 1243 771107 or email: enquiries@summersdale.com.

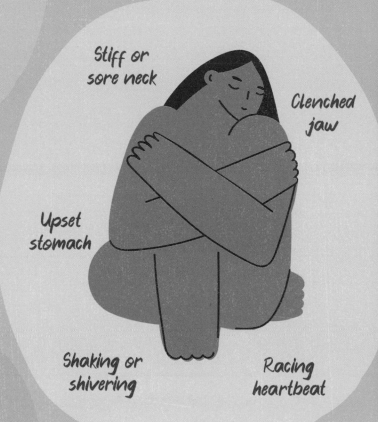

Symptoms of stress:

Stiff or
sore neck

Clenched
jaw

Upset
stomach

Shaking or
shivering

Racing
heartbeat

Little steps...

Tentative steps...

Half steps...

Are all steps in the right direction

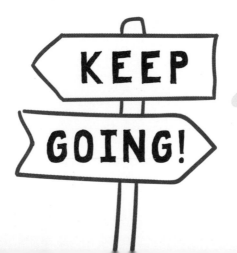

Stay strong
through your pain,
grow flowers
from it.

RUPI KAUR

Simple scripts
TO ASK FOR SUPPORT

I'm feeling low today. I don't want to talk about it but could you send me something cute/funny/delicious to distract me?

I'm not feeling great. Can we arrange a time to talk?

It's been a tough week. Can we schedule something fun?

CHECK IN WITH YOUR EMOTIONAL SELF TODAY

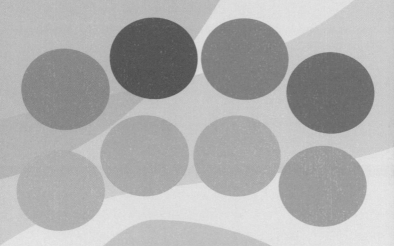

Which colour
best reflects your mood?
Track how your mood-colour
changes over the course of a week.
You may notice that certain days are
always certain mood-colours. Consider
why that may be and what affects your
mood – negatively or positively.

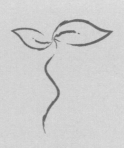

GROW
A LITTLE
EVERY
DAY

THE PARTS OF YOU THAT ARE WORTHY OF
LOVE:

The good friend part

The kind to animals part

The sense of humour part

The talented part

The anxious part

The wants to do better part

The sometimes feeling sad part

The needs some time to yourself part

THE PARTS OF YOU THAT ARE
NOT WORTHY OF LOVE:

Nope. Nada. Nothing. All of you is worthy of love.

*No sunbeam
ever lies.*

E. E. CUMMINGS

YOU deserve
loveliness

Sunrises

Dew

Hot coffee

Fresh sheets

Scented candles

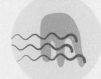

Favourite songs

Old books

Moonlight

Compliments

negative self-talk and ways to identify burnout, this is a book that will take you by the hand and say what you need to hear. Even if what you need to hear is, "It's okay to wrap yourself in a duvet burrito for the day." This handy guide is designed to be opened up when you feel like you're shutting down. So go ahead – it's time to leave the blue moods behind and experience the full rainbow.

INTRODUCTION

We need the little things in life as much as the big moments. A break in the clouds, a hug at the right moment, the small voice in the back of our heads that says, "I can do this." These moments are the rich soil in which we grow our self-esteem, our resilience and our relish for life.

These pages are filled with dozens of these little moments. From simple ideas to lift your spirits and self-care rituals to strategies to combat

THINGS TO DO

WHEN YOU'RE

Feeling Blue

FELICITY HART

IMAGE CREDITS

HOTLINES

Those who feel very low and would like to talk to someone straight away can reach help via hotlines. Although some hotlines are called "suicide prevention lines", they can also help with crises, provide instant support and connect you with the resources you need.

https://www.samaritans.org/
https://suicidepreventionlifeline.org/
https://www.prevent-suicide.org.uk/
https://www.thetrevorproject.org/

CHARITY INSIGHT

One of the symptoms of many types of blues is that you second guess yourself. You may doubt your judgement or fear that feeling vulnerable leaves you vulnerable. Or, you may simply want to know as much information as possible about an organization before you reach out to them. Here are a few resources that can help you have confidence in those who may assist you.

https://www.charitynavigator.org/
https://www.charityclarity.org.uk/

RESOURCES

Sometimes we need a little extra help. Speaking to a professional or accessing resources can be the assistance we need to navigate the issues at hand. Think of them as new members of "Team You"! They may be one-off features or a loan for the season. The help you need is available.

MENTAL HEALTH

Learn more about caring for your mental health and how to access resources and infrastructure to your benefit.

https://www.mind.org.uk/

https://mhanational.org/

ANXIETY

Looking for help with managing your anxiety? There are charities that specialize in providing support and resources.

https://www.anxietyuk.org.uk/

https://adaa.org/

CONCLUSION

Good luck on your mental health journey.
Remember that even the strongest person
can have sad days, or moments of frustration,
or times when they feel like that they've not
succeeded. These moments do not define you.
Well done for everything you've achieved and
will continue to achieve.

Keep doing the best for yourself, whether that is
using the self-care techniques and pick-me-up
moments in this book, or reaching out to your
loved ones and support network.

Even at your most flawed, you're perfect. Even
when you feel broken, you're whole. You're
brilliant, unique and worthy. Keep going.

Love yourself

A LITTLE BIT
MORE TODAY

YOUR SONG
DESERVES
TO BE
HEARD

USE THE BUDDY SYSTEM

Loved ones can help us navigate social situations we find challenging. Next time you're feeling concerned about an upcoming event, ask a buddy to:

Investigate a location ahead of time

Intercept and divert awkward questions

Practise some socializing scripts

Schedule a half-time "check-in"

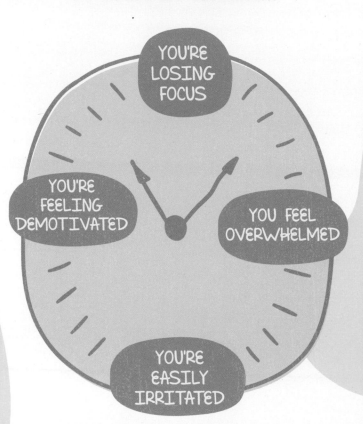

Skin care IS SELF-CARE

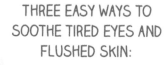

THREE EASY WAYS TO
SOOTHE TIRED EYES AND
FLUSHED SKIN:

1. Keep a gel mask in the fridge. Apply it to your sore face and lie back. Let the coolness refresh your skin.

2. Mist your face with a soothing rose mist spray. This provides an instant pick-me-up. Carry a travel-sized bottle so it can provide quick relief when on the go.

3. Run your wrists under cold water. The delicate skin at your pulse points allows the water to quickly cool your body. The perfect remedy for feeling puffy.

While there's
life there's hope.

MIGUEL DE CERVANTES

THINGS THAT
ARE FRAGILE
CAN ALSO BE
BEAUTIFUL

QUICKTORIES
(6 SPEEDY VICTORIES)

Change your pillowcase

Drink a glass of water

Open a window

Give yourself a compliment

Look at a cute pic

Deep breath in, deep breath out

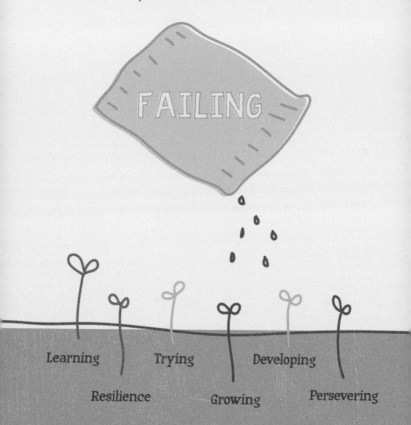

Don't judge
each day by the
harvest you reap
but by the seeds that
you plant.

ROBERT LOUIS STEVENSON

YOUR
TIMELINE

You are here

Moment of joy

Delicious food

Good times with friends

Beautiful view

There is still so much yet to come

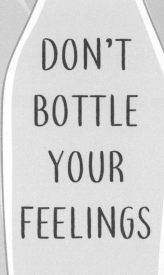

DON'T
BOTTLE
YOUR
FEELINGS

Talk to yourself like you would to someone you love.

BRENÉ BROWN

Mess

Tidying can create a lot of *mess*
before you achieve *results*

Life is like that too

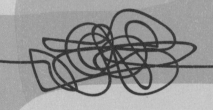

Sometimes things get *messy*
before they get *better*

But they do get *better*

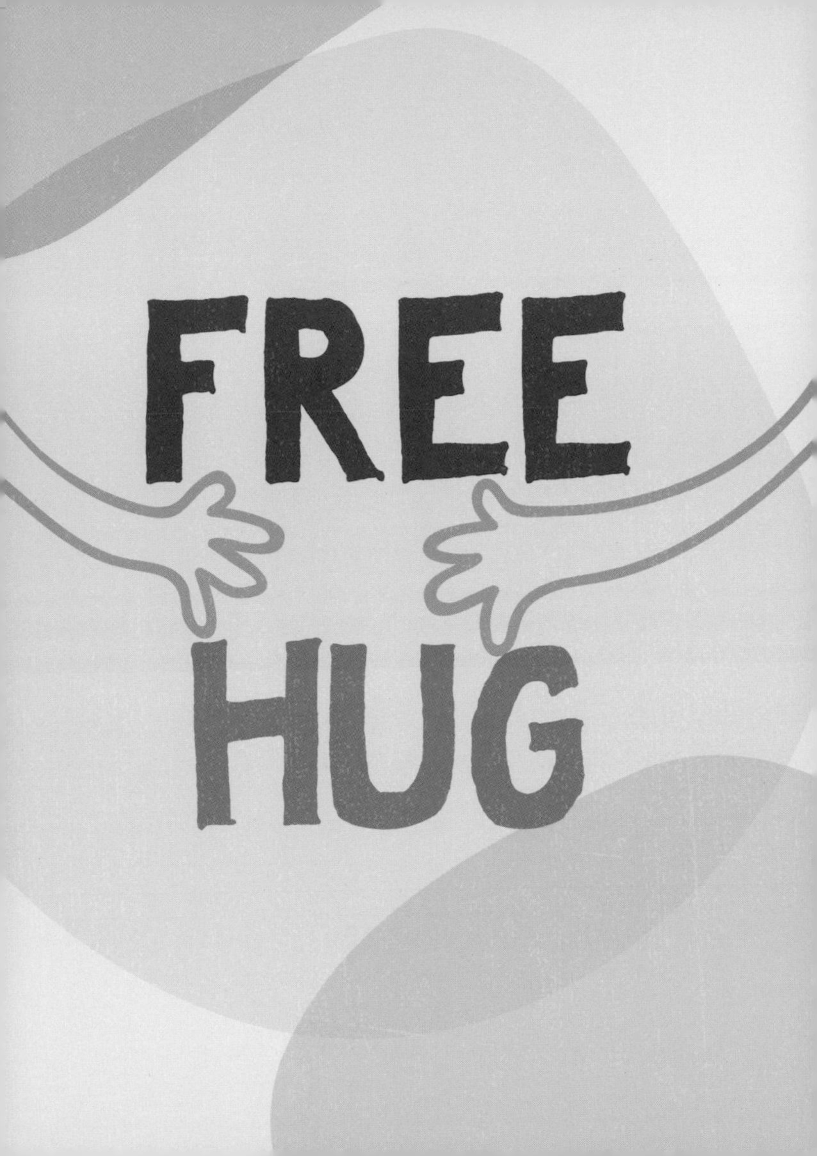
FREE
HUG

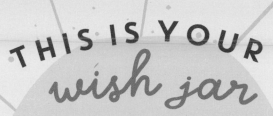

THIS IS YOUR
wish jar

**FULL OF THINGS TO MAKE
YOU FEEL BETTER. TODAY,
THE WISH JAR CONTAINS...**

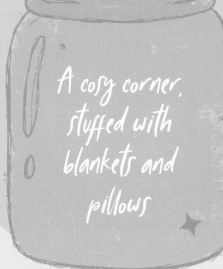

A cosy corner,
stuffed with
blankets and
pillows

Here's a cup of

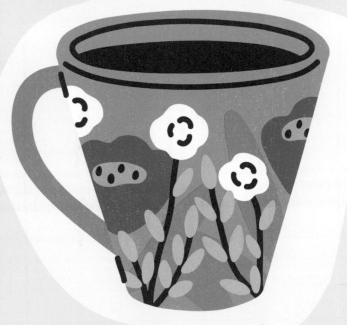

positive-tea

BEFORE YOU GO TO

sleep tonight

CLOSE THE TABS IN

your head

HOW TO
REST EASY

✷
**Create a
bedtime
routine**

✷
**Reserve your
bedroom for
sleep**

✷
**Dim the
lights**

✷
**Change
your sheets
regularly**

✷
**Ban
electronic
devices**

✷
**Keep your
bed clear of
clutter**

And to tired limbs and
over-busy thoughts,
Inviting sleep and soft
forgetfulness.

WILLIAM WORDSWORTH

HAPPY HOME

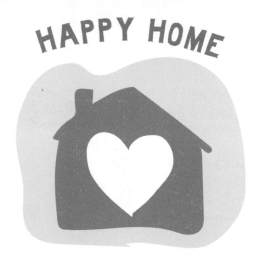

Blue wavelengths – commonly known as blue light – are emitted by electronic devices, such as smartphone screens. Research has found that exposure to this light during the evening can disrupt our sleeping rhythms. A good night's sleep is an important tool in the mental health toolkit. Incorporate a period of winding down in your bedtime ritual. Turn off your screens half an hour before you are ready to sleep. Keep your bedroom free of devices and resist the temptation to scroll as you lie in bed.

I am the master
of my fate,
I am the captain
of my soul.

WILLIAM ERNEST HENLEY

LIST OF VICTORIES AND SUCCESSES

Getting out of bed

Showering

Opening your curtains/blinds

Preparing a filling meal

Messaging a loved one

Going outside for 5 minutes

Saying one kind thing to yourself

Noticing a beautiful thing

BODY CHECK-IN

Unclench your jaw

Drop your shoulders

Breathe out deeply

Stand up straight

Uncross your arms

TODAY IS A
self-care
DAY

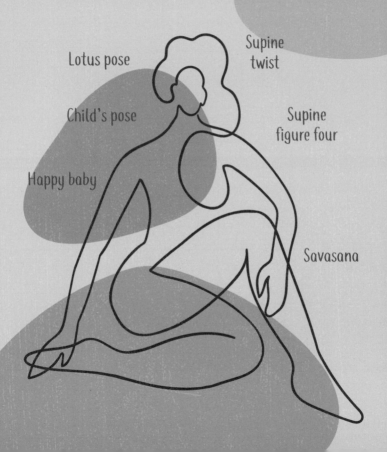

Restorative yoga poses to calm, centre and unwind

Lotus pose

Supine twist

Child's pose

Supine figure four

Happy baby

Savasana

Expecting the worst, you look, and instead, here's the joyful face you've been wanting to see.

RUMI

SELF-CARE BENTO BOX

Eating foods that slowly release energy can help regulate your mood. Pack yourself an anxiety-reducing bento box.

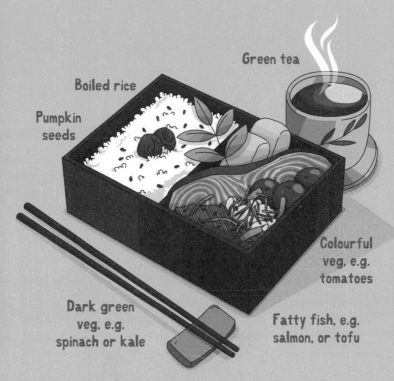

Green tea

Boiled rice

Pumpkin seeds

Colourful veg, e.g. tomatoes

Dark green veg, e.g. spinach or kale

Fatty fish, e.g. salmon, or tofu

HAPPY HOME

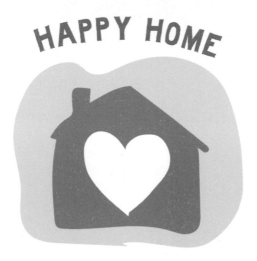

Feeling anxious, depressed or blue can heighten your awareness of your surroundings – to your detriment. Noises that are simply a fact of life, like people laughing or music drifting in from elsewhere, can start to cause flares of temper and frustration. Make your home a little sanctuary by playing calming music. Or, if you are feeling really overstimulated, try white noise. White noise is a mixture of sound frequencies and studies show that it can have a calming effect.

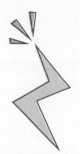

RECHARGE
YOUR
SOUL

RITUALS

Sometimes you need the support of your own best ally – Past You! Past You knows what you find challenging and can help you prepare for the day ahead.

Set a nightly "helpful half hour" to tackle the things you struggle with:

- Prep your bag, or put things you know you'll need by the door.

- Set reminders for errands that you know you'll forget.

- Set an alarm for 20 minutes before you need to leave (and maybe for 10 minutes before, too!).

HEY YOU!
BE KIND TO YOURSELF

CATASTROPHIZING TRIAGE

Now you've identified what you're experiencing, it's time to tackle some of the symptoms. Triage is used in medicine to swiftly organize and treat patients. Here triage takes the form of simple solutions that can quickly and directly alleviate your symptoms.

Schedule time to worry and **don't exceed** that time

Acknowledge that the source of your feelings is hypothetical

Identify **possible triggers**

Practise **mindfulness**

Keep a **log** of your predictions...

... and **refer back** to see how few come true

Signs you're experiencing...
CATASTROPHIZING

Catastrophizing is the act of spinning out a hypothetical bad scenario into the worst-possible case. For example, when planning on meeting a friend, you might start to plan what to do if you get lost. Then the scenario escalates – what if you're late, you miss each other and your friendship ends? Catastrophizing can be a symptom of other challenges, such as anxiety or depression, or simply an issue in itself.

Assuming the worst will happen	"Practising" conversations...
Overplanning and overpreparing for routine activities	... and feeling upset or angry at their outcome
Seeking external validation and reassurance	Blaming yourself for factors out of your control

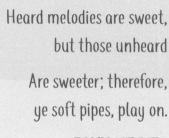

Heard melodies are sweet,
but those unheard

Are sweeter; therefore,
ye soft pipes, play on.

JOHN KEATS

POSITIVE
SELF-TALK
SPINNER

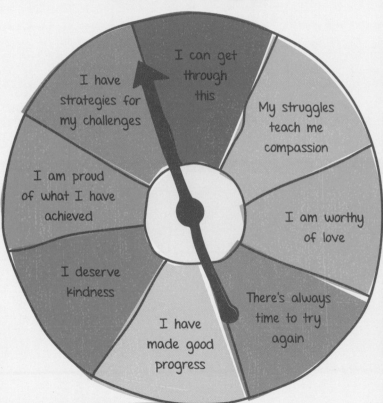

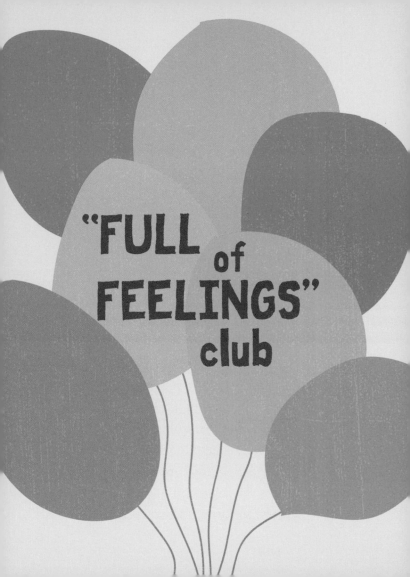

SOMETIMES WHEN WE MEDITATE, OUR MINDS WANDER

Here is a happy little thought

Simply acknowledge the thought

Hello happy little thought

And return your focus to your breathing, letting the thought drift away

Goodbye thought

MEDITATION KIT

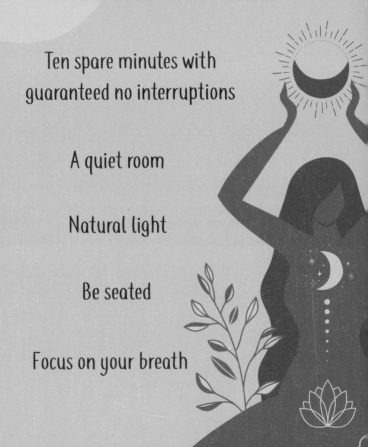

Ten spare minutes with
guaranteed no interruptions

A quiet room

Natural light

Be seated

Focus on your breath

There's always a rainbow —
sometimes you just have to find it

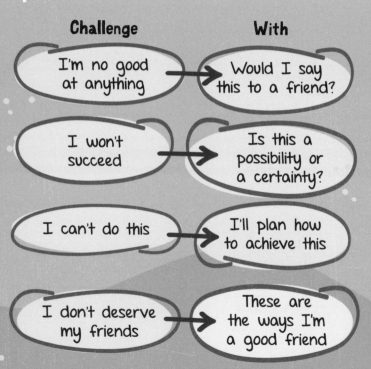

Don't wish away
your cracked past,
your crooked toes.

MARTY McCONNELL

SELF-LOATHING TRIAGE

Now you've identified what you're experiencing, it's time to tackle some of the symptoms. Triage is used in medicine to swiftly organize and treat patients. Here triage takes the form of simple solutions that can quickly and directly alleviate your symptoms.

Identify your **triggers**

Practise **positive self-talk** (even when you don't want to)

Forgive - and forget - **your mistakes**

Talk to **yourself** like you'd talk to your **friends**

Journal your **good choices** and **actions**

Signs you're experiencing...
SELF-LOATHING

Self-esteem is the foundation on which many healthy behaviours are built. However, it can be hard to build self-esteem when your biggest critic is yourself. How can you know when your opinion of yourself has slipped from "firm but fair" to being a bit of a bully? Here are some examples of how self-loathing can manifest itself.

Inability to believe good things about yourself

Negative self-talk

Hyperfixation on your mistakes or "bad" decisions

Believing feelings are facts

Giving up before you begin

Unfavourable comparisons to others

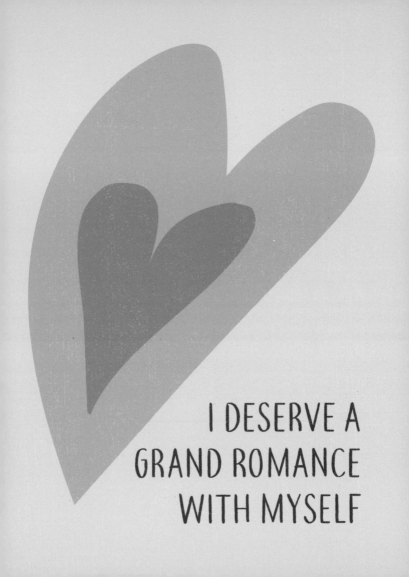

I DESERVE A
GRAND ROMANCE
WITH MYSELF

THIS IS YOUR
wish jar

FULL OF THINGS TO MAKE YOU FEEL BETTER. TODAY, THE WISH JAR CONTAINS...

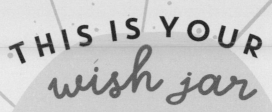

A quiet evening curled up watching anything you want

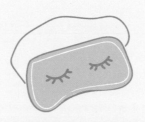

FEELING TIRED BUT STILL INSPIRED

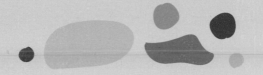

MANIFESTING A
good day

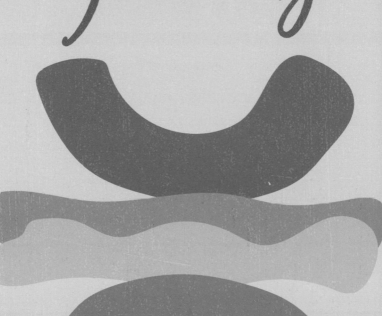

THE "BE LESS FLAKY" PLAN

Sometimes it's easier to just dip. If you've got into the habit of avoiding events and now want to start coming out of your shell, here's how.

Practical

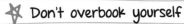

⭐ Don't overbook yourself

⭐ Suggest an alternative date instead of "squeezing" plans in

Emotional

⭐ Be honest with yourself –
do you want to say yes?

⭐ Be honest with others –
it's okay to say no

Technological

⭐ Use reminders, apps and diaries

⭐ As soon as you make a plan,
make a note or diarize it

Hope is the thing
with feathers
That perches in
the soul.

EMILY DICKINSON

SITUATIONAL LONELINESS

Living away from home

May be travelling
or relocating

Unable to easily see
or talk to loved ones

Close friends and
family live far away

CHRONIC LONELINESS

Has been lonely
for a long time

Struggling to make
personal connections

Feels burnt out by
social interactions

TYPES OF LONELINESS

EMOTIONAL LONELINESS

Has loved ones and
a social circle

Still feels lonely

Loneliness not tied to circumstances
but comes from within

SOCIAL LONELINESS

Feels lonely in social situations

Can be socially awkward

Intimidated by large groups
or meeting new people

Doesn't feel lonely in
one-on-one situations

LONELINESS TRIAGE

Now you've identified what you're experiencing, it's time to tackle some of the symptoms. Triage is used in medicine to swiftly organize and treat patients. Here triage takes the form of simple solutions that can quickly and directly alleviate your symptoms.

Cut down on **social media**

Identify the **root cause** of your loneliness

Meet a friend in person or talk on the phone

Talk to a **professional** about it

Join a **hobby group**

Get some **fresh air and exercise**

Signs you're experiencing...
LONELINESS

Loneliness doesn't only hit when you're alone. You can feel lonely when with friends or family – or even, as the old saying goes, in the middle of a crowd. Loneliness doesn't always manifest in expected ways. Sure, you may ache for some companionship, or a real connection. But you could also be feeling lonely if you're experiencing:

Outsized reactions to disruptions and disappointments

Restless or disrupted sleep

An increased desire for material possessions

Binge watching TV or playing games

Overeating

Substituting social warmth for physical warmth, such as long showers

Sensory self-care

Mindfully eat your favourite snack

Stand barefoot on grass

Look to the horizon

Walk past a bakery and inhale the scents

Listen to a joyful song

YOU ARE
enough

HAPPY HOME

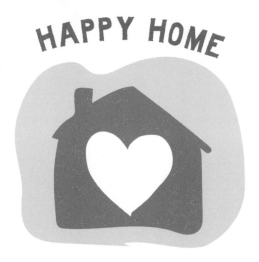

Are you struggling with feelings of restlessness, anxiety or sensory distraction? A weighted blanket can alleviate symptoms related to these challenges. Weighted blankets contain evenly distributed balls or pellets that cause the blanket to apply pressure. To some, this pressure has the effect of feeling like you're being hugged or swaddled, creating a sense of calm. If you enjoy physical contact, it could be worth investing in a weighted blanket for times of need.

Hair care
IS SELF-CARE

THREE EASY WAYS TO CARE FOR YOUR HAIR:

1. Gently brush or comb out all the tangles. It doesn't matter how they got there, they're gone now.

2. Massage your scalp during your next shampoo.

3. Apply a conditioning mask. Your hair deserves nourishment too.

I am larger,
better than I thought;
I did not know I held
so much goodness.

WALT WHITMAN

YOU DON'T HAVE TO APOLOGIZE FOR...

Having a bad day

Wanting something different

Needing your space

Taking up space

Prioritizing yourself

You are NOT
your MISTAKES

YOU

YOUR
MISTAKES

CALL SOMEONE
WHO LOVES YOU

YOU'VE GOT TO

nourish

TO

flourish

WHAT'S YOUR SUCCULENT MOOD TODAY?

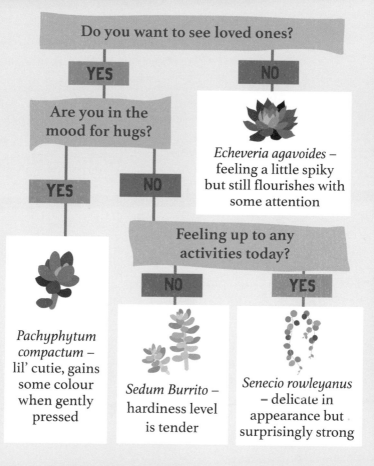

Do you want to see loved ones?

YES **NO**

Are you in the mood for hugs?

Echeveria agavoides – feeling a little spiky but still flourishes with some attention

YES **NO**

Feeling up to any activities today?

NO **YES**

Pachyphytum compactum – lil' cutie, gains some colour when gently pressed

Sedum Burrito – hardiness level is tender

Senecio rowleyanus – delicate in appearance but surprisingly strong

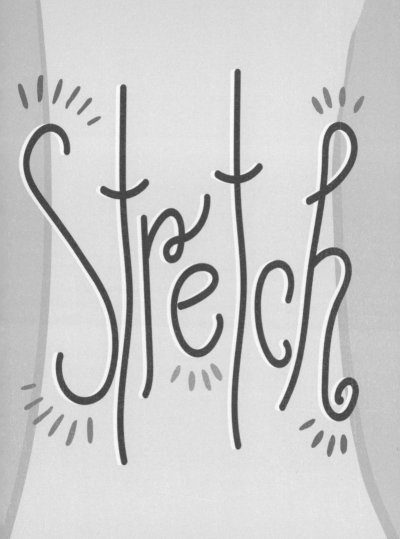

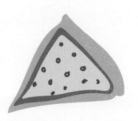

SOMETIMES
SELF-CARE
IS PIZZA
AND NAPS

RITUALS

Why self-care, anyway? How can baths or sheet masks have a positive impact on your mental health? When you have the blues, your self-worth can drop and your daily routine can be one of surviving, instead of thriving. Self-care is about treating yourself like you matter (you do) and helping your mind through maintaining your health.

Apply a sheet mask: be mindful in the moment, breathing deeply and noting the cool sensation of the mask on your skin. Your skin will feel refreshed and smooth, and embodiments of stress, such as dry skin, will be soothed.

There must be quite
a few things that a
hot bath won't cure,
but I don't know
many of them.

SYLVIA PLATH

DEAR self,
I love
YOU

HECK YEAH! FACE MASKS

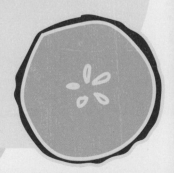

ANXIETY TRIAGE

Now you've identified what you're experiencing, it's time to tackle some of the symptoms. Triage is used in medicine to swiftly organize and treat patients. Here triage takes the form of simple solutions that can quickly and directly alleviate your symptoms.

Try some breathing exercises

Acknowledge that your worries may be **rooted** in **anxiety**

Journal regularly to **identify triggers**

Create **healthy** **sleep** routines

Talk to a **medical** **professional**

Signs you're experiencing...
ANXIETY

Anxiety is a persistent feeling of unease or dread. Most people will feel anxious about something in their lifetime, such as new or unusual situations like a job interview. However, sometimes anxiety can be a more persistent issue which has an impact on our mental or physical welfare. Common symptoms of anxiety include:

Fixation on negative hypothetical situations

Sweaty palms

A feeling of dread

Restlessness

A tight chest

An upset stomach

IF you wouldn't
say it to OTHERS

DON'T say it
to yourself

THINGS TO THROW IN THE BIN

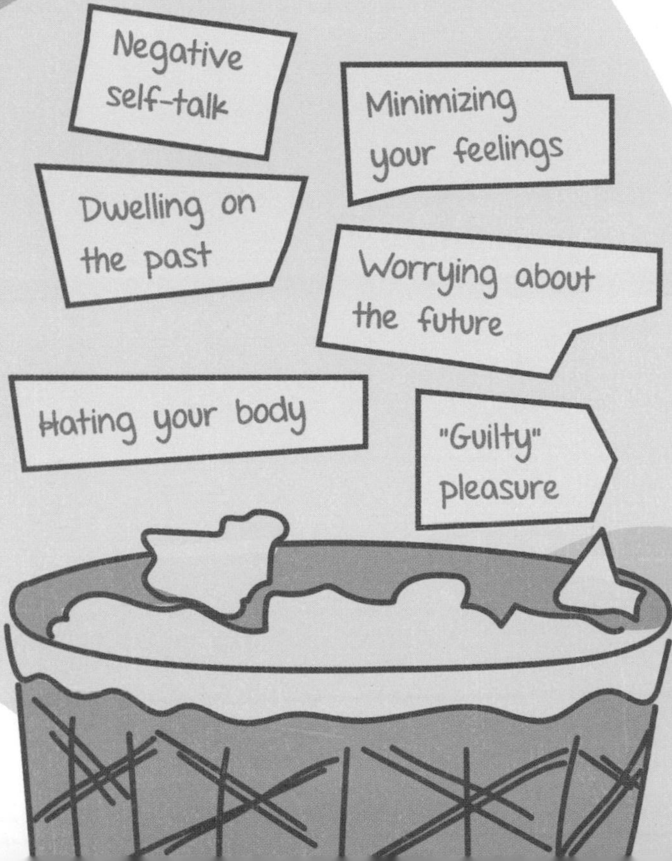

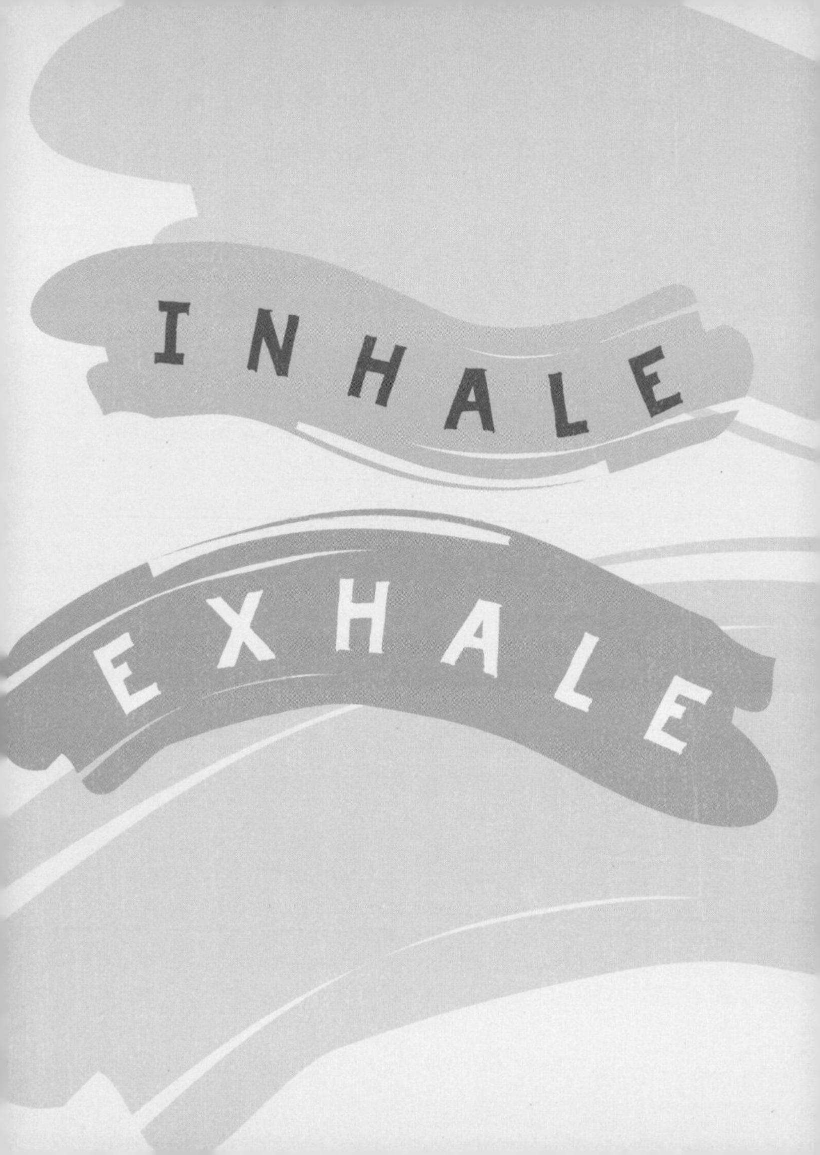
INHALE
EXHALE

Colour-slide your mood — feel the full spectrum

What does my future hold?

A HUG
Ice cream
A cute dog Flowers
SUNSHINE
A bath

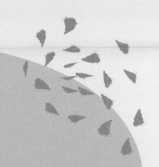

New hope is fairer
than an old regret.

ELLA WHEELER WILCOX

IF YOUR AIMS
AND ASPIRATIONS
ARE FEELING OUT OF REACH,
LOOK BEHIND YOU. YOU'LL SEE
HOW FAR YOU'VE TRAVELLED.

EVEN

dope

PEOPLE HAVE

nope

DAYS

It's okay to...

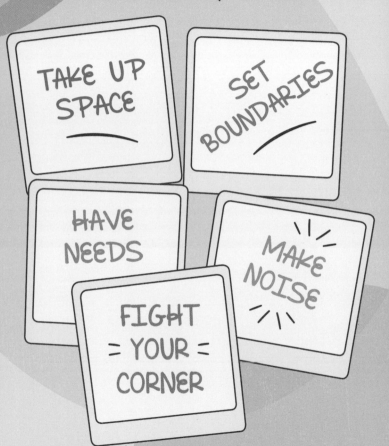

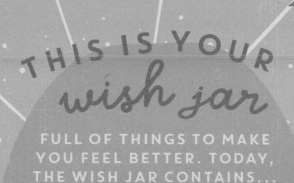

THIS IS YOUR
wish jar

FULL OF THINGS TO MAKE
YOU FEEL BETTER. TODAY,
THE WISH JAR CONTAINS...

*Your favourite
song, played at
full volume*

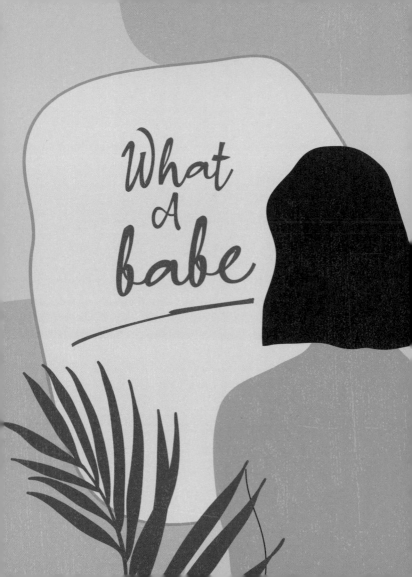

THIS IS YOUR
" *no more guilty pleasures* "
T I C K E T

YOU CAN ENJOY
PLEASURE
FOR ITS OWN
SAKE

HAPPY HOME

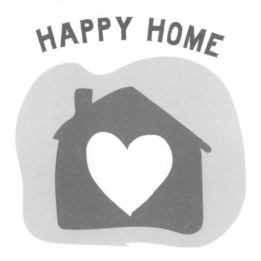

Natural light is a mood booster. Increase your exposure to natural light in your home. Simply opening the curtains when you feel like shutting out the world can help lift your mood. Not every home has the "perfect" set-up for catching the rays. Create your own DIY sun-worshipping spot by bringing blankets, cushions, plants and books to the sunniest space in your home. Who cares if you're chilling in the hallway?

Feeling good > being normal

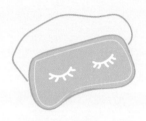

ADULTS
NEED
A NAP
TOO

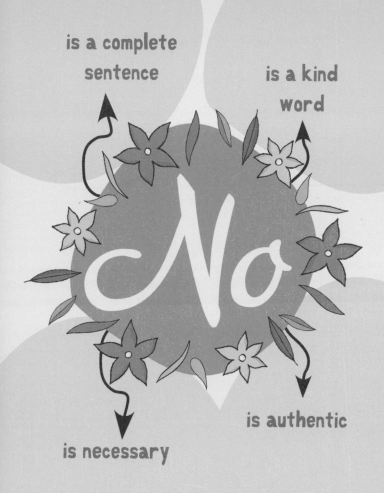

ESTABLISHING BOUNDARIES
is self-care

BURNOUT TRIAGE

Now you've identified what you're experiencing, it's time to tackle some of the symptoms. Triage is used in medicine to swiftly organize and treat patients. Here triage takes the form of simple solutions that can quickly and directly alleviate your symptoms.

Acknowledge that you feel **overwhelmed**

Say **no** to new tasks

Identify which responsibilities are **top priority**

Delegate, defer or **drop** low priority tasks

Signs you're experiencing...
BURNOUT

Burnout is the feeling of physical and mental exhaustion caused by being overloaded. Workplace stress is a common cause of burnout. The pressure to "have it all" outside of work can also result in burnout, as people attempt to juggle the demands of being present for friends and family, socializing, participating in hobbies, volunteering, self-development or upskilling, maintaining fitness and other "healthy" habits. Common symptoms of burnout include:

Feeling demotivated and disengaged

Stress

Task avoidance

Forgetfulness

Anxiety

Increased escapist activities

Hard times
require furious
dancing.

ALICE WALKER

CRYING IS A VALID WAY TO EXPRESS YOUR EMOTIONS

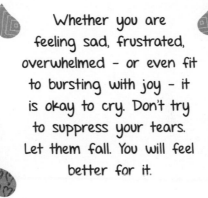

Whether you are feeling sad, frustrated, overwhelmed - or even fit to bursting with joy - it is okay to cry. Don't try to suppress your tears. Let them fall. You will feel better for it.

NOT

perfect

JUST TRYING MY

best

Don't focus
on everything
you aren't

FOCUS ON
EVERYTHING
YOU ARE

RITUALS

Journaling can be a useful daily ritual to help track and manage your mood. Jot down the events of the day and your feelings. Over time you may be able to track connections between certain events and feelings, identifying triggers. Journaling can also be a way to develop positive habits. For example, if you are prone to negative thought cycles at the end of the day, then include journaling as part of your bedtime ritual, writing down three good things that occurred that day.

I need

S P A C E

to grow

H.A.L.T!

Do you need help identifying the source of unexpected negative emotions? Recognizing the root of a bad feeling can stop it blossoming into bad behaviour. Pause, take a breath and H.A.L.T. Are you feeling:

Hungry?

Angry?

Lonely?

Tired?

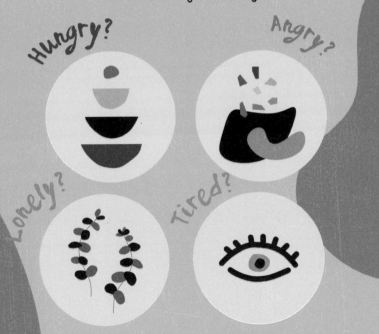

Crucial to finding the way is this: there is no beginning or end. You must make your own map.

JOY HARJO

BLUE spaces

... ARE THE AREAS AROUND
NATURAL BODIES OF WATER.

THIS INCLUDES
STREAMS, RIVERS,
LAKES, WATERFALLS,
SEAS AND THE OCEAN.

SPENDING TIME IN GREEN OR BLUE
SPACES CAN HAVE A POSITIVE
IMPACT ON YOUR MENTAL HEALTH.

GREEN spaces

... ARE AREAS FILLED WITH PLANTS AND VEGETATION.

THIS INCLUDES PARKS, GARDENS, NATURE RESERVES, FORESTS,

HILLS, MOUNTAINS, GARDENS AND ALLOTMENTS.

Some plants need lots of light

 Some plants need plenty of shade

 Some plants like chalky soil

 Some plants prefer clay soil

 Plants have different needs

 So do humans

 And that's okay

Be your own plant mama

Water yourself – hydration is important

Cut back unnecessary "foliage"

Nourish yourself

Plant yourself where there's space to grow

Get plenty of natural light

It's okay to outgrow others

SWITCH

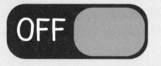

REPLACE
toxic positivity
WITH
healthy validation

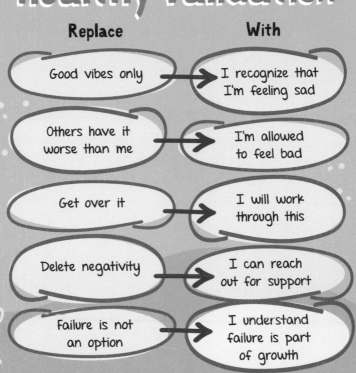

Replace	With
Good vibes only	I recognize that I'm feeling sad
Others have it worse than me	I'm allowed to feel bad
Get over it	I will work through this
Delete negativity	I can reach out for support
Failure is not an option	I understand failure is part of growth

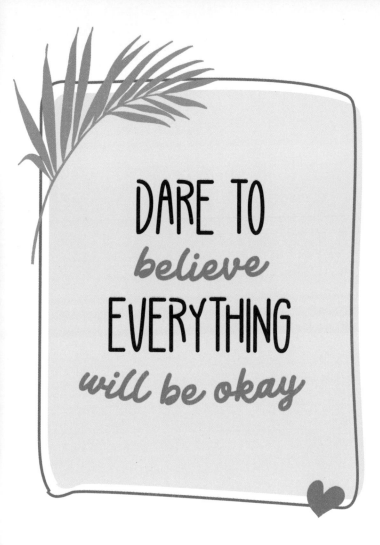

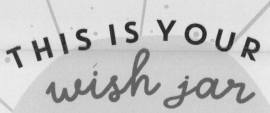

THIS IS YOUR
wish jar

FULL OF THINGS TO MAKE
YOU FEEL BETTER. TODAY,
THE WISH JAR CONTAINS...

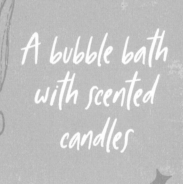

A bubble bath
with scented
candles

SELF-CARE IS:

- Eating healthily
- Exercising
- Drinking herbal tea
- Regular sleep
- Stretching

Self-care can also be...

- A big slice of cake
- Naps
- Wearing your comfy sweater three days in a row
- Watching your favourite films

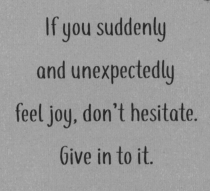

If you suddenly

and unexpectedly

feel joy, don't hesitate.

Give in to it.

MARY OLIVER

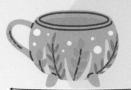
Break down tasks
into smaller steps

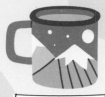
Relax your
muscles

CUPS OF
DE-STRESS
Tea

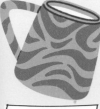
Meditate

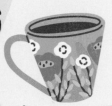
Ask for help

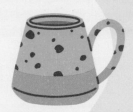
Log off
social media

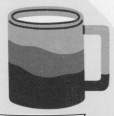
Take regular
breaks